Gluten Free Autoimm

A Beginner's 4-Week Step-by-Step Guide With Curated Recipes

Introduction
    Power of Diet
    Diet in Autoimmune Diseases
    What You'll Discover from this Guide:

Chapter 1: Gluten
    Where is gluten found?
    What is it composed of?
    Common Complaints
    Pathophysiology
    Common Diseases Associated with Gluten
    Other Diseases Associated with Gluten
    Sex-Biased: Women

Chapter 2: AutoImmune Diseases
    What are autoimmune diseases?
        1. Genetic Predisposition
            Females > Males
            Ethnic Groups
        2. Exposure to Infections and Chemicals
        3. Hygiene Hypothesis
        4. Western Diet
    Common Autoimmune Diseases
    Cost of Autoimmune Diseases

Chapter 3: Benefits of GFD
    In Autoimmune Diseases
    In General

Chapter 4: How do you practice a gluten-free diet?

Week 1: Remove all sources of gluten from your kitchen and medicine cabinets.

Week 2: Just Fresh Produce and Meat

Week 3: Practice Distinguishing Gluten-Free Products

Week 4: Join Support Groups and ASK Questions

Chapter 5: Conclusion

Gluten- Free Recipes

Day 1: Pad Thai

Day 2: Pecan and Maple Salmon

Day 3: Pork Chops, Carrots and Buckwheat

Day 4: Cacao Nibs, Figs, and Oats

Day 5: Cobb Salad

Day 6: Shredded Chicken Chili

Day 7: Shrimp Avocado Salad

References

Disclaimer

By reading this disclaimer, you are accepting the terms of the disclaimer in full. If you disagree with this disclaimer, please do not read the book. The content in this book is provided for informational and educational purposes only.

This book is not intended to be a substitute for the original work of this diet plan. At most, this book is intended to be a beginner's supplement to the original work for this diet plan and never acts as a direct substitute. This book is an overview, review, and commentary on the facts of that diet plan.

All product names, diet plans, or names used in this book are for identification purposes only and are property of their respective owners. The use of these names does not imply endorsement. All other trademarks cited herein are the property of their respective owners.

None of the information in this book should be accepted as an independent medical or other professional advice.

Introduction

"The doctor of the future will no longer treat the human frame with drugs, but rather will cure and prevent disease with nutrition."
- Thomas Edison

The Power of Diet

Food is the only constant thing we introduce in our bodies on a daily basis— giving it the power to influence our normal physiology and biochemistry in a number of ways.

While its original purpose was to support the growth and function of the human body, it is now one of the major culprits for chronic diseases.

We have undermined what our diet can do to the human body. Allowing ourselves to be unaware of how it can even modify the anatomy of our intestines and brains.

We succumb to the aggressive marketing of the food industry, confusing us with a plethora of food choices. With our guards down and without being mindful of what we are absorbing into our system, we are granting it authority over our mental and physical health.

Perhaps, by enlightening ourselves with healthier options and intentionally planning our meals, we can be more in control of our health. We can lessen chronic diseases and reduce the need for pharmaceutical drugs. And maybe prevent future pandemics from happening.

Diet in Autoimmune Diseases

A suitable diet varies for every individual.

It depends on your BMI, level of activity, presence of deficiencies, convenience, palate preference, ideal weight, etc.

However, when it comes to autoimmune diseases, it is more than advised by studies to eliminate foods that overstimulate the immune system.

Hence, the Gluten-Free Diet (GFD).

Although there is no hard evidence (yet) that can claim that GFD promotes nutritional health benefits, there are a number of studies that cannot deny associations between GFD and alleviation of symptoms in autoimmune diseases. Most especially in Celiac Disease, Gluten Ataxia, Dermatitis Herpetiformis, and Type 1 Diabetes Mellitus.

If you want to take control of your body, and not the other way around, here is a manual to provide you with basic information about autoimmune diseases and how it can be affected by gluten. And hopefully, encourage you to be more intentional with your diet or nutritional biochemistry.

What You'll Discover from this Guide:

1. The hidden dangers of gluten in autoimmune diseases
2. Basic knowledge on autoimmune diseases
3. Reversal of symptoms from GFD
4. Tips on how to practice GFD more effectively
5. Sample GFD for beginners

Chapter 1: Gluten

Where is gluten found?

"Gluten" was derived from a Latin term, which means "glue".

It is the "glue" that keeps the food together and is responsible for the dough formation in flour— making bread tasty and easy to make.

Gluten is basically found in wheat, barley, rye, and spelt.

More specifically in:[1]

Grains	Processed Grain-Based Products	Other Foods & Beverages
Whole wheat	Crackers	Barley malt
Wheat bran	Bread	Malt vinegar
Barley	Breadcrumbs	Soy sauce
Rye	Pasta	Certain salad dressings
Triticale	Seitan	Sauces
Spelt	Wheat- containing	Gravy thickened with flour
Kamut	soba noodles	Bouillon |
Couscous	Some veggie	Some broths
Farro	burgers	Certain spice blends
Semolina	Cookies	Flavored chips
Bulgur	Pastries	Beer
Farina		Certain kinds of wine
Einkorn		
Wheat germ		
Cracked wheat		
Matzo		
Mir (wheat + rye)		

[1] Hill, A. (2020, January 13). What Is Gluten? Definition, Foods, and Side Effects. Retrieved May 2020, from https://www.healthline.com/nutrition/what-is-gluten

Gluten may also be found in pharmaceutical drugs, supplements, cosmetics and hygiene products.[2]

What is it composed of?

Gluten is a protein composed of 45- 50% polymeric glutenins and 50- 55% monomeric gliadins in a family called prolamins.[3]

Gliadin gives the bread the ability to rise during baking, and glutenin is responsible for the dough's elasticity.

These prolamins are composed of a long sequence of peptide molecules such as proline and glutamine, which is difficult for our digestive system to break down.

One kind of wheat can contain forty-five (45) different gliadins. Each having a different set of properties contributing to the different reactions to the human body.

---

[2] Cohen, I., Day, A., & Shaoul, R. (2019, January 1). Gluten in Celiac Disease — More or Less? Retrieved May 17, 2020, from https://www.ncbi.nlm.nih.gov/pmc/articles/PMC6363368/

[3] Day, L. (2011). Wheat gluten: production, properties and application. Retrieved 2020, from https://www.sciencedirect.com/science/article/pii/B9781845697587500101

Some of these properties can activate the innate immune response making gluten disadvantageous to autoimmune diseases.[4]

---

[4] Niland, B., & Cash, B. (2018, February). Health Benefits and Adverse Effects of a Gluten-Free Diet in Non–Celiac Disease Patients. Retrieved May 2020, from https://www.ncbi.nlm.nih.gov/pmc/articles/PMC5866307/

Common Complaints

The common complaints associated with gluten are the following:[56]

Gastrointestinal	Skin	Neurologic
• Loose bowel stools/ Diarrhea • Vomiting • Abdominal pain • Feeling of bloatedness • Constipation • Blood-streaked stool	• Inflammatory papules and vesicles on the scalp, forearms, elbows, knees, and buttocks	• Poor coordination of the extremities • Ocular problems • Gait disturbance • Tingling sensation on the extremities • Slurred or slow speech

[5] Hill, A. (2020, January 13). What Is Gluten? Definition, Foods, and Side Effects. Retrieved May 2020, from https://www.healthline.com/nutrition/what-is-gluten

[6] Akhondi, H. (2020, March 24). Gluten And Associated Medical Problems - StatPearls - NCBI Bookshelf. Retrieved May 2020, from https://www.ncbi.nlm.nih.gov/books/NBK538505/

Pathophysiology

There are theories that suggest that the human intestine has not fully adapted yet to accommodate the biochemical structure and length of gluten-derived peptides, leading to a couple of modifications in one's normal physiology.[7]

These are:

1. Leaky Gut

There is a protein called "Zonulin" that allows the in-and-out of molecules through the intestinal epithelial barrier— making it possible for nutrients to be absorbed into the bloodstream.

---

[7] Niland, B., & Cash, B. (2018, February). Health Benefits and Adverse Effects of a Gluten-Free Diet in Non–Celiac Disease Patients. Retrieved May 2020, from https://www.ncbi.nlm.nih.gov/pmc/articles/PMC5866307/

However, with an increase in levels of Zonulin from gluten intake and autoimmune diseases, the permeability of the barrier is also increased—overriding the normal passage and absorption of molecules.[8][9] Eventually, allowing bacteria and toxins to make it through the bloodstream.[10]

2. Inflammation

Immune responses stimulated by gluten intake introduce autoantibodies in different tissues or organs.

One common example is inflammation in the small intestine.

Normally, compounds from our diet are absorbed via the outermost layer of the small intestine where food digestion is completed.

---

[8] Diag, P. B. (2018, April). What is zonulin? – Creative Diagnostics Blog. Retrieved May 2020, from https://www.creative-diagnostics.com/blog/index.php/what-is-zonulin/

[9] pubmeddev. (2012, February). Leaky gut and autoimmune diseases. - PubMed - NCBI. Retrieved May 2020, from https://www.ncbi.nlm.nih.gov/pubmed/22109896

[10] "Is Leaky Gut Syndrome a Real Condition? An Unbiased Look." 2 Feb. 2017, https://www.healthline.com/nutrition/is-leaky-gut-real. Accessed 20 May. 2020.

Upon gluten intake, inflammatory factors locally infiltrate the intestinal mucosa disturbing the normal absorption of nutrients.[11]

3. Cross-Reactivity

The protein structure of some of the components of wheat and milk are similar to the structure of our self- antigens.

Cross-reactivity happens when antibodies mistakenly target our self- antigens, instead of the antigenic substances from wheat and milk, and develop an immune response.[12] [13]

---

[11] Niland, B., & Cash, B. (2018, February). Health Benefits and Adverse Effects of a Gluten-Free Diet in Non–Celiac Disease Patients. Retrieved May 2020, from https://www.ncbi.nlm.nih.gov/pmc/articles/PMC5866307/

[12] pubmeddev. (2015). Molecular mimicry as a mechanism for food immune reactivities and autoimmunity. - PubMed - NCBI. Retrieved May 2020, from https://www.ncbi.nlm.nih.gov/pubmed/25599184

[13] Fairweather, D., & Rose, N. (2004, November 1). Women and Autoimmune Diseases. Retrieved May 18, 2020, from https://www.ncbi.nlm.nih.gov/pmc/articles/PMC3328995/

Common Diseases Associated with Gluten

The most common diseases associated with gluten-sensitivity are:

1. Celiac Disease (Autoimmune Disease)

It is a gluten-induced disease causing damage to the anatomy of the intestines. Associated with specific genes such as HLA-DQ2 and HLA-DQ8, and autoantibodies (anti-tissue transglutaminase and antiendomysial). Manifesting with both gastrointestinal and extraintestinal symptoms like fatigue and dizziness.[14]

Upon gluten consumption, the villi of the intestines are anatomically damaged causing intestinal permeability. Subsequently, affecting nutrient absorption and developing gastrointestinal and extra- intestinal symptoms.

---

[14] pubmeddev. (2017, August). Celiac Disease and Nonceliac Gluten Sensitivity: A Review. - PubMed - NCBI. Retrieved May 15, 2020, from https://www.ncbi.nlm.nih.gov/pubmed/28810029

Some of the gastrointestinal symptoms include "abdominal pain, diarrhea, unintentional weight loss, and constipation." Whereas the extra-intestinal symptoms are "iron deficiency anemia, reduced bone density or osteoporosis, infertility, miscarriage, skin rash (dermatitis herpetiformis), depression, elevated liver enzymes, neuropathy, and headaches."[15]

2. Non- Celiac Gluten Sensitivity

NCGS is a gluten-induced disorder similar to Celiac Disease. But without the anatomical changes in the intestines. Where reversal of symptoms is noted after gluten withdrawal.[16]

---

[15] Jones, A. (2017, May 1). The Gluten-Free Diet: Fad or Necessity? Retrieved May 18, 2020, from
https://www.ncbi.nlm.nih.gov/pmc/articles/PMC5439366/

[16] pubmeddev. (2017, August). Celiac Disease and Nonceliac Gluten Sensitivity: A Review. - PubMed - NCBI. Retrieved May 15, 2020, from
https://www.ncbi.nlm.nih.gov/pubmed/28810029

Other Diseases Associated with Gluten

1. Gluten Ataxia

It is commonly seen in patients who are in their 50's to 60's. Manifesting symptoms of poor coordination and balance, and a tingling sensation in the extremities.

This occurs when antibodies, from gluten intake, infiltrate the cerebellum and attack the purkinje fibers causing degeneration and atrophy.[17] [18]

2. Dermatitis Herpetiformis

This is usually associated with Celiac Disease and Non- Celiac Gluten Sensitivity.

---

[17] Niland, B., & Cash, B. (2018, February). Health Benefits and Adverse Effects of a Gluten-Free Diet in Non–Celiac Disease Patients. Retrieved May 2020, from https://www.ncbi.nlm.nih.gov/pmc/articles/PMC5866307/

[18] Akhondi, H. (2020, March 24). Gluten And Associated Medical Problems - StatPearls - NCBI Bookshelf. Retrieved May 2020, from https://www.ncbi.nlm.nih.gov/books/NBK538505/

But instead of finding IgA deposits on the gut, they are seen in the epidermis. Manifesting with inflamed papules and vesicles with moderate to severe itchiness on the scalp, forearms, buttocks and knees.[19]

3. Wheat or Grain Allergy

The IgE deposits from gluten intake result in allergic reactions such as skin atopy, oropharyngeal edema, and cardiovascular collapse.

Others may be non-IgE mediated developing enterocolitis (inflammation of the small and large intestines), proctitis (inflammation of the rectum), and enteropathy (intestinal disease).

Wherein, both cases are common in children.[20]

[19] Akhondi, H. (2020, March 24). Gluten And Associated Medical Problems - StatPearls - NCBI Bookshelf. Retrieved May 2020, from https://www.ncbi.nlm.nih.gov/books/NBK538505/

[20] Akhondi, H. (2020, March 24). Gluten And Associated Medical Problems - StatPearls - NCBI Bookshelf. Retrieved May 2020, from https://www.ncbi.nlm.nih.gov/books/NBK538505/

Sex-Biased: Women

With gluten- containing diet, estrogen levels are known to increase, inhibiting the cytochrome P-450 3A4 system. Which plays an important role in the metabolism of medicines and other compounds.

Thereby, increasing the risk of toxicity from drugs and other compounds in the body.

This is why women with chronic estrogen dominance are encouraged to get Anti- Gliadin Antibody Testing to check for any gluten sensitivity.[21]

---

[21] Rakel, D. (2012). *Integrative Medicine: Expert Consult Premium Edition - Enhanced Online Features and Print (Rakel, Integrative Medicine)* (3rd ed.). Philadelphia, USA: Elsevier Saunders.

Chapter 2: Autoimmune Diseases

What are autoimmune diseases?

The normal human physiology has an innate immune system that defends the body from foreign invaders that are suspected to cause harm.

However, there are instances; wherein, this default protective system malfunctions. Eventually, targeting harmless cells and organs in our body.

Hence, the term "Autoimmune."

Although the etiology remains to be a mystery. Studies have shown associations with the following:

1. Genetic Predisposition

Females > Males

Autoimmune diseases are the third most common disease in the US. Affecting 8% of the population (14- 22 million people). Majority of which are women (78%) in their child bearing age.[22]

Some studies have linked the increased risk in women with their more pronounced inflammatory responses.

This sex-bias can be explained by the direct control of estrogen and androgens over immune cells such as TH1 and TH2-- increasing the production of pro inflammatory cytokines.[23]

Ethnic Groups

Autoimmune diseases are seen to cluster among ethnic groups.

The genes responsible for apoptosis, or self-termination of immune responses, could be an inherited factor.

---

[22] Fairweather, D., & Rose, N. (2004, November 1). Women and Autoimmune Diseases. Retrieved May 18, 2020, from https://www.ncbi.nlm.nih.gov/pmc/articles/PMC3328995/

[23] Fairweather, D., & Rose, N. (2004, November 1). Women and Autoimmune Diseases. Retrieved May 18, 2020, from https://www.ncbi.nlm.nih.gov/pmc/articles/PMC3328995/

However, the risk of developing an autoimmune disease is only 30-35% accounted for by genetic predisposition.[24]

2. Exposure to Infections and Chemicals

Studies have shown that, with or without genetic predisposition, autoimmune diseases are mostly triggered by drugs, viruses, bacteria, and other environmental factors.[25]

Perhaps, a constant exposure to these factors make the body more defensive even to self-antigens.[26]

3. Hygiene Hypothesis

[24] Fairweather, D., & Rose, N. (2004, November 1). Women and Autoimmune Diseases. Retrieved May 18, 2020, from
https://www.ncbi.nlm.nih.gov/pmc/articles/PMC3328995/

[25] Autoimmune disease. (2014, January 1). Retrieved May 2020, from
https://www.sciencedirect.com/science/article/pii/B9780702054013000187

[26] Mackay, I. (1998, January 1). Autoimmune Diseases. Retrieved May 18, 2020, from
https://www.sciencedirect.com/science/article/pii/B0122267656000761

In contrast to the previous point, some studies also show that a low-level of exposure to pathogens make the body more susceptible to infections. Allowing the body to be less capable of combating infections.

Which is why, once exposed in an unusual environment, the overreaction of the immune system occurs.[27]

4. Western Diet

Western diet refers to high cholesterol, high fat, and high sugar food.

Consumption of high fat in western diet promotes excess White Adipose Tissue (WAT), which plays a role in the activation of pro-inflammatory cytokines.

[27] Okada, H., Kuhn, C., Feillet, H., & Bach, J.-F. (2010, April 1). The 'hygiene hypothesis' for autoimmune and allergic diseases: an update. Retrieved May 16, 2020, from https://www.ncbi.nlm.nih.gov/pmc/articles/PMC2841828/

Common Autoimmune Diseases

According to American Autoimmune Related Diseases Association (ARDA), there are more than 100 diseases under this category[28]— affecting the "endocrine system, connective tissue, gastrointestinal tract, heart, skin, and kidneys."[29]

They vary depending on the auto-antibody profile, clinical manifestations, and tissue affected.

These are the common autoimmune diseases:[30]

1. Type 1 DM
2. Rheumatoid Arthritis
3. Psoriasis/ Psoriatric Arthritis
4. Multiple Sclerosis
5. Systemic Lupus Erythematosus
6. Inflammatory Bowel Disease
7. Addison's Disease
8. Graves' Disease
9. Sjogren's Syndrome

---

[28] Autoimmune Disease List – AARDA. (2018). Retrieved May 18, 2020, from https://www.aarda.org/diseaselist/

[29] Fairweather, D., & Rose, N. (2004, November 1). Women and Autoimmune Diseases. Retrieved May 18, 2020, from https://www.ncbi.nlm.nih.gov/pmc/articles/PMC3328995/

[30] Watson, S. (2019, March 26). Autoimmune Diseases: Types, Symptoms, Causes, and More. Retrieved May 15, 2020, from https://www.healthline.com/health/autoimmune-disorders

10. Hashimoto's Thyroiditis

Cost of Autoimmune Diseases

Having an autoimmune disease is quite taxing-- from diagnosing to its management.

In order to diagnose an autoimmune disease, a series of tests are needed to:

1. Determine whether it is a systemic disease affecting multiple organs
2. Determine whether it is affecting a single organ
3. Identify the "disease relevant autoantibody" for a more specific diagnosis[31]

A few examples for initial testing include:[32]
- Serum immunoglobulin A (IgA)
- anti-tissue transglutaminase (TTG) antibodies
- C-reactive protein (CRP)
- ESR (erythrocyte sedimentation rate),
- ANA (antinuclear antibodies)

Whereas, examples of specific tests include:[33]

[31] Fairweather, D., & Rose, N. (2004, November 1). Women and Autoimmune Diseases. Retrieved May 18, 2020, from https://www.ncbi.nlm.nih.gov/pmc/articles/PMC3328995/
[32] Jones, A. (2017, May 1). The Gluten-Free Diet: Fad or Necessity? Retrieved May 18, 2020, from https://www.ncbi.nlm.nih.gov/pmc/articles/PMC5439366/
[33] Mackay, I. (1998, January 1). Autoimmune Diseases. Retrieved May 18, 2020, from

- Anti- globulin reaction in hemolytic anemia
- Autoantibodies to:
  - ☐ Acetylcholine receptor in Myasthenia Gravis
  - ☐ Adrenal cortical cells in Addison's Disease
  - ☐ dsDNA in SLE
  - ☐ Mitochondrial pyruvate dehydrogenase enzyme complexes in primary biliary cirrhosis
  - ☐ Combination of nuclei and F actin in type 1 autoimmune hepatitis

Others even require regular testing as deemed necessary by the consulting physician.

In addition to this, managing the symptoms with immunosuppressant medications are also costly.

https://www.sciencedirect.com/science/article/pii/B012226765 6000761

Chapter 3: Benefits of GFD

Since there are over 80 kinds of autoimmune diseases and a few more on the waiting list to be approved under the same category, the autoimmune diseases that will be discussed in this chapter are those that are related to gluten and have been well-studied.

In Autoimmune Diseases

Studies on gluten-free diet have shown associations with improvement in malabsorption, nutritional deficiencies, symptoms, and co-morbidities in autoimmune diseases.[34]

By elimination of gluten from diet alone, a significant reduction of circulating proinflammatory mediators have been noted.

---

[34] Reilly, N. (2016, August). The Gluten-Free Diet: Recognizing Fact, Fiction, and Fad. Retrieved May 17, 2020, from https://secure.jbs.elsevierhealth.com/action/cookieAbsent?code =null

Celiac Disease & Type 1 DM

The decrease in local immune response on the small intestine addresses the malabsorption by subsequently reversing anatomical changes created by gluten-induced inflammation.[35] Leading to an improvement in gastrointestinal and extra-intestinal symptoms. [36] Such as diarrhea, steatorrhea, unintentional weight loss, developmental delay, and anemia.[37]

Eventually, easing vitamin and mineral deficiencies such as vitamin B12, calcium iron, folate, vitamin D, magnesium, carotenoids, thiamin, copper, selenium, etc.[38]

For instance, a strict gluten-free diet is the only treatment for Celiac Disease. Wherein daily gluten intake should be within 10- 50mg only.[39]

[35] Akhondi, H. (2020, March 24). Gluten And Associated Medical Problems - StatPearls - NCBI Bookshelf. Retrieved May 2020, from https://www.ncbi.nlm.nih.gov/books/NBK538505/

[36] Jones, A. (2017, May 1). The Gluten-Free Diet: Fad or Necessity? Retrieved May 18, 2020, from https://www.ncbi.nlm.nih.gov/pmc/articles/PMC5439366/

[37] Zuvarox, T. (2020, January 8). Malabsorption Syndromes - StatPearls - NCBI Bookshelf. Retrieved May 19, 2020, from https://www.ncbi.nlm.nih.gov/books/NBK553106/

[38] Zuvarox, T. (2020, January 8). Malabsorption Syndromes - StatPearls - NCBI Bookshelf. Retrieved May 19, 2020, from https://www.ncbi.nlm.nih.gov/books/NBK553106/

[39] Cohen, I., Day, A., & Shaoul, R. (2019, January 1). Gluten in Celiac Disease — More or Less? Retrieved May 17, 2020, from https://www.ncbi.nlm.nih.gov/pmc/articles/PMC6363368/

In addition to this, there have been studies that show "reduced cholesterol levels, lower A1C values, and lower rates of retinopathy and nephropathy" in patients with Celiac Disease and Type I DM.[40]

Due to a possible reduction in antibodies responsible for the islet cell destruction in Type 1 DM, gluten-free diet has improved HbA1c levels in children with Type 1 DM.[41]

Dermatitis Herpetiformis

GFD has also decreased cutaneous IgA deposits in Dermatitis Herpetiformis.[42]

A long-term (8 to 18 months) practice of strict gluten-free diet has resulted in a decrease of medication in 70% to 100% of patients with Dermatitis Herpetiformis. And 40% to 70% were able to withdraw medications completely after 2 years or more.[43]

---

[40] Jones, A. (2017, May 1). The Gluten-Free Diet: Fad or Necessity? Retrieved May 18, 2020, from https://www.ncbi.nlm.nih.gov/pmc/articles/PMC5439366/

[41] Svensson, J., Sildorf, S. M., Pipper, C. B., Kyvsgaard, J. N., Bøjstrup, J., Pociot, F. M., … Buschard, K. (2016). Potential beneficial effects of a gluten-free diet in newly diagnosed children with type 1 diabetes: a pilot study. *SpringerPlus*, 5(1), 1–8. https://doi.org/10.1186/s40064-016-2641-3

[42] Dietary management of dermatitis herpetiformis. - PubMed - NCBI. (1987, October). Retrieved May 19, 2020, from https://www.ncbi.nlm.nih.gov/pubmed/3662571

[43] Dietary management of dermatitis herpetiformis. - PubMed -

Gluten Ataxia

And lastly for Gluten Ataxia, neurologic deficits can be slowed down or prevented from progressing with GFD. But since the damage is on the cerebellum, the anatomical impairment is not reversible.[44]

NCBI. (1987, October). Retrieved May 19, 2020, from https://www.ncbi.nlm.nih.gov/pubmed/3662571

[44] Akhondi, H. (2020, March 24). Gluten And Associated Medical Problems - StatPearls - NCBI Bookshelf. Retrieved May 2020, from https://www.ncbi.nlm.nih.gov/books/NBK538505/

In General

Although, there is no hard data to support the theory that GFD has promising health benefits for <u>healthy</u> individuals. A survey was done back in 2009 to 2014, where one-year of GFD resulted in weight loss, lower waist circumference, and an increase in high-density lipoprotein (HDL).[45]

As for women suffering from chronic pelvic pain and Endometriosis, six to twelve months of GFD has shown significant relief from pain in two studies.[46]

Whereas among athletes, improvement in self-reported gastrointestinal symptoms was noted.[47]

---

[45] Niland, B., & Cash, B. (2018, February). Health Benefits and Adverse Effects of a Gluten-Free Diet in Non–Celiac Disease Patients. Retrieved May 2020, from https://www.ncbi.nlm.nih.gov/pmc/articles/PMC5866307/
[46] Niland, B., & Cash, B. (2018, February). Health Benefits and Adverse Effects of a Gluten-Free Diet in Non–Celiac Disease Patients. Retrieved May 2020, from https://www.ncbi.nlm.nih.gov/pmc/articles/PMC5866307/
[47] Niland, B., & Cash, B. (2018, February). Health Benefits and Adverse Effects of a Gluten-Free Diet in Non–Celiac Disease Patients. Retrieved May 2020, from https://www.ncbi.nlm.nih.gov/pmc/articles/PMC5866307/

Chapter 4: How do you practice a gluten-free diet?

"Control your perceptions.
Direct your actions properly.
Willingly accept what's outside your control."
- Ryan Holiday

We know how difficult it is to practice GFD. So here is a step-by-step guide to help you get used to GFD.

Do not fret. Be hopeful and stay strong in the fact that it only takes 21 days (or 3 weeks) to develop a habit.

Step-by-Step Guide on How to Practice GFD

Week 1: Remove All Sources of Gluten from Your Kitchen and Medicine Cabinets

Dispose or donate all foods and ingredients containing gluten. Such as:

1. Wheat-based foods
2. Barley
3. Rye
4. Triticale (Cross between wheat and rye)
5. Malt
6. Brewer's yeast

Also, do not forget to clean out your medicine cabinet and remove gluten-containing cosmetics, toothpaste, vitamins, supplements, and pharmaceutical drugs. Since wheat starch is usually used in tablets and capsules as a binding agent.[48]

---

[48] "What medicines and non-food products have gluten? - WebMD." https://www.webmd.com/digestive-disorders/celiac-disease/qa/what-medicines-and-nonfood-products-have-gluten. Accessed 22 May. 2020.

If you are extremely sensitive to the smallest amount of gluten, we encourage you to replace regularly used kitchen tools like your frying pan and cooking utensils.[49]

Here is a checklist to avoid cross-contamination with your gluten-free food:[50]

- ☐ Replace the toaster and only use it for gluten-free bread
- ☐ Replace cooking pans with stainless steel
- ☐ Replace ovenware or place a foil or parchment paper
- ☐ Replace dishwashing materials
- ☐ Purchase a new non-porous chopping board
- ☐ Have a separate storage area for gluten-free food

During this period, you can start introducing gluten-free food into your diet at least once a day. And practice cooking them yourself at home.

[49] 8 Easy Steps to Kick Gluten to the Curb … Permanently. (2020, April 7). Retrieved May 22, 2020, from
https://www.verywellfit.com/how-to-go-gluten-free-563172

[50] The Beginners Guide to Going Gluten Free | Vida sin gluten. (n.d.). Retrieved May 23, 2020, from
https://www.schaer.com/en-us/a/how-go-gluten-free-beginners

Week 2: Just Fresh Produce and Meat

At this point, it is not safe yet to explore processed gluten-free foods. Since you have yet to learn how to identify what is *actually* gluten-free from what *claims* to be gluten-free.

To keep it simple, stick first with meat and fresh produce. (They are usually found on the sides of the supermarket.)

Plan your meals ahead of time and make a grocery list that you promise to stick to while doing your grocery shopping. This will also help in avoiding unnecessary calories from alternatives and from developing nutritional deficiencies.[51]

If you have existing comorbid diseases and nutritional deficiencies, we encourage you to seek consultation with a dietician first before finalizing your grocery list.

Once in the grocery, skip the sections for junk and processed food. Not only will you get to save money, but you will also be able to save up so much time.

---

[51] EatingWell. (2019, May 1). Starting a Gluten-Free Diet: A Guide for Beginners. Retrieved May 15, 2020, from http://www.eatingwell.com/article/288542/starting-a-gluten-free-diet-a-guide-for-beginners/

Week 3: Practice Distinguishing Gluten-Free Products

When ready, you can now explore the processed food section in the supermarket. And make time to look for "gluten-free" labels by the FDA.

There are ingredients and products in the market that claim to be gluten-free but still contain small amounts of gluten.

According to the Food and Drug Administration (FDA) under the Food Allergen Labeling and Consumer Protection Act of 2004 (FALCPA), foods labeled "gluten-free" should only contain 20 parts per million (ppm) gluten per kilogram of food or less.[52]

Look closely and double check if there is any hint of gluten in the list of ingredients. The common ones would be milk, eggs, and wheat.

Since you still need to watch your nutrition, stay away from complicated labels. Usually, the longer the label, the more processed it is.

The following are some examples of gluten-free food and ingredients:[53]

---

[52] Food labeling: gluten-free labeling of foods. Final rule. - PubMed - NCBI. (2013, August). Retrieved May 18, 2020, from https://www.ncbi.nlm.nih.gov/pubmed/23923139

Basics	Grains and Starch-containing:	Beverages:
1. Fruits 2. Vegetables 3. Meat and poultry 4. Fish and seafood 5. Dairy 6. Beans, legumes, and nuts	1. Rice 2. Cassava 3. Corn 4. Potato 5. Soy 6. Tapioca 7. Sorghum 8. Quinoa 9. Millet 10. Buckwheat groats 11. Amaranth 12. Arrowroot 13. Teff 14. Flax 15. Chia 16. Yucca 17. Gluten-free oats 18. Nut flour	Most beverages are gluten-free. But it's safer to always check the labels. Avoid "beers, ales, lagers, malt beverages and malt vinegars."

[53] Gluten-Free Foods. (n.d.-b). Retrieved May 18, 2020, from https://celiac.org/gluten-free-living/gluten-free-foods/

More of this list in "Gluten Free Food List | IBS Diet"[54]

For more guidelines on the recommended daily intake, you may refer to:
Nutrient Recommendations : Dietary Reference Intakes (DRI)[55]

[54] Gluten Free Food List | IBS Diets. (n.d.-b). Retrieved May 18, 2020, from https://www.ibsdiets.org/ibs/gluten-free-food-list/

[55] Nutrient Recommendations: Dietary Reference Intakes (DRI). (n.d.). Retrieved May 18, 2020, from https://ods.od.nih.gov/Health_Information/Dietary_Reference_Intakes.aspx

Week 4: Join Support Groups and ASK Questions

In order to sustain this new lifestyle, it always helps to have a support group that can be your source of encouragement.

They can provide you with creative recipes that can make gluten-free food more delectable. And they can give you the best tips on where to eat and where to buy goods in your community.

Week 5: Eat Out and Socialize

Once confident enough that you can identify gluten ingredients accurately, you can now start eating out in restaurants.

Always ask if the meal you are about to order is gluten-free. Or if the staff is not knowledgeable enough, ask for the ingredients. It is always better to ask and be sure, than assume and regret later on.

And of course, practicing GFD should not hinder you from eating out with friends and family. You can always suggest your restaurant choices or bring a home-cooked meal that you can share-- they might even enjoy it and influence them to convert.

Chapter 5: Conclusion

"The definition of disease rests, rather, on the specific disabilities caused by an incongruity between an individual's genetic endowment and his or her current environment— between a mutation, the circumstances of a person's existence, and his or her goals for survival or success. It is not mutation that ultimately causes disease, but mismatch."
- Siddhartha Mukherjee

GFD is not fully advised for the general population due to its lack of evidence in improving one's nutritional profile— lower fiber, iron, zinc, and potassium.[56]

Although there is no data supporting health benefits in healthy individuals, multiple studies are able to associate gluten-free diet with significant relief from recurring symptoms in autoimmune diseases. Combined with proper planning of meals with a registered dietician in order to avoid nutritional deficiencies.

---

[56] Jones, A. (2017, May 1). The Gluten-Free Diet: Fad or Necessity? Retrieved May 18, 2020, from
https://www.ncbi.nlm.nih.gov/pmc/articles/PMC5439366/

This supports the theory that genes only account for 33% of one's physiology, where 77% is attributed to one's environmental factors.[57]

Hence, having a genetic predisposition for an autoimmune disease is not the final dictum. It takes environmental variables— diet, lifestyle, nutrition— to turn on the switch for autoimmunity to push through.

You may have the producer to start a play. But you also need a handful of staff to make the play actually happen— your director, writer, stage crew, logistics, costume designer, etc.

With a proper diet, you can restore function and optimize your life.

The following section contains Gluten-Free Recipes that you can follow until you are able to get the hang of GFD.

Enjoy!

---

[57] Day, L. (2011). Wheat gluten: production, properties and application. Retrieved 2020, from https://www.sciencedirect.com/science/article/pii/B978184569 7587500101

Gluten- Free Recipes

Day 1: Pad Thai

Carbohydrates: 52%
Fat: 34%
Protein: 14%

INGREDIENTS

5 ounces pad Thai rice noodles

3 tablespoons vegetable oil

1 large egg, room temperature

6 medium shrimp, peeled, deveined (optional)

2 tablespoons 1x½x⅛-inch slices pressed tofu (bean curd)

1 tablespoon sweet preserved shredded radish, rinsed, chopped into 1-inch pieces

1 cup bean sprouts

5 tablespoons tamarind water, or 2 tablespoons plus 1 teaspoon tamarind paste mixed with 2 tablespoons plus 1 teaspoon water

1½ tablespoons (or more) Thai fish sauce (nam pla)

1½ tablespoons simple syrup, preferably made with palm sugar

4 garlic chives, 2 cut into 1-inch pieces

½ teaspoon ground dried Thai chiles, divided

2 tablespoons crushed roasted, unsalted peanuts, divided

2 lime wedges

INSTRUCTIONS

1. Place noodles in a large bowl; pour hot water over to cover.
2. Let soak until tender but don't make it mushy, 5–10 minutes.
3. Drain; set aside.
4. Heat vegetable oil in a wok or large skillet over medium-high heat.
5. Add egg; stir until barely set, about 30 seconds. Add shrimp, if using.
6. Cook, stirring, until shrimp and egg are almost cooked through, 2–3 minutes.
7. Add tofu and radish; cook for 30 seconds. Add noodles and cook for 1 minute.
8. Stir in sprouts. Add tamarind water, fish sauce, and simple syrup and stir-fry until sauce is absorbed by noodles and noodles are well coated, about 1 minute.
9. Stir in chopped garlic chives. Add 1/4 tsp. ground chiles and 1 Tbsp. peanuts and toss well.
10. Transfer to serving plates.
11. Garnish with remaining 1/4 tsp. ground chiles, 1 Tbsp. peanuts, and lime wedges.

Day 2: Pecan and Maple Salmon

Carbohydrates: 12%
Fat: 59%
Protein: 28%

INGREDIENTS
1 tablespoon apple cider vinegar
1 teaspoon smoked paprika
1/2 teaspoon chipotle pepper powder
1/2 teaspoon onion powder
Add all ingredients to list

INSTRUCTIONS
1. Place salmon fillets on a baking sheet and season with salt and black pepper.
2. Combine pecans, maple syrup, vinegar, paprika, chipotle powder, and onion powder in a food processor; pulse until texture is crumbly.
3. Spoon pecan mixture on top of each salmon fillet, coating the entire top surface.
4. Refrigerate coated salmon, uncovered, for 2 to 3 hours.
5. Pre-heat oven to 425 degrees F (220 degrees C).
6. Bake salmon in the preheated oven until fish flakes easily with a fork, 12 to 14 minutes.

Day 3: Pork Chops, Carrots and Buckwheat

Carbohydrates: 15%
Fat: 58%
Protein: 44%

INGREDIENTS
1 orange
1½ pound carrots, scrubbed, halved lengthwise, cut into 2" pieces
1 garlic clove finely grated
2 tablespoons olive oil, plus more
Kosher salt
2 teaspoons fresh lime juice, plus more
¾ cup pearled buckwheat groats
1 tablespoon vegetable oil
2 1"-thick bone-in pork shoulder chops (about 8–10 oz. each)
3 tablespoons unsalted butter, divided
¼ cup dill sprigs
Aleppo or Urfa pepper or crushed red pepper flakes

INSTRUCTIONS
1. Cut all peel and white pith from orange; discard.
2. Working over a small bowl, cut along sides of membranes to release segments; squeeze in juice as well.
3. Preheat the oven to 450°. Toss carrots, garlic, and 2 Tbsp. olive oil on a rimmed baking sheet; season with salt.

4. Roast, tossing once, until tender and browned, 15–20 minutes.
5. While carrots are still hot, add orange segments and juice and 2 tsp. lime juice and toss to coat. Set aside.
6. Meanwhile, cook buckwheat in a large saucepan of boiling salted water until tender but not falling apart, 10–15 minutes.
7. Drain; rinse under cold water. Spread out on a baking sheet and let dry
8. Heat vegetable oil in a large heavy skillet over high.
9. Season pork with salt and cook until browned but still pink in the center, about 4 minutes per side.
10. Add 1 Tbsp. butter and spoon over chops, turning once, 1 minute. Transfer to a cutting board and let rest for 10 minutes.
11. Meanwhile, add cooled buckwheat and remaining 2 Tbsp. butter to skillet; season with salt.
12. Cook, tossing often, until grains are toasted and some are crisp, about 5 minutes. Drain on paper towels.
13. Slice pork; toss dill into buckwheat.
14. Serve buckwheat and carrots with slices of pork, drizzled with lime juice and olive oil and sprinkled with Aleppo pepper.

Day 4: Cacao Nibs, Figs, and Oats

Carbohydrates: 75%
Fat: 12%
Protein: 13%

INGREDIENTS
1½ cups Big Batch of Steel-Cut Oat
2 tablespoons cacao nibs
6 dried Turkish figs, 4 chopped, 2 sliced
Almond milk

INSTRUCTIONS
1. Combine cooked oats and ¼ cup water in a medium saucepan over medium-low heat.
2. Stir in cacao nibs and chopped figs and continue to cook, stirring occasionally, until oats are warmed through, about 3 minutes.
3. Thin to desired consistency with almond milk, and serve topped with sliced figs.

Day 5: Cobb Salad

Carbohydrates: 10%
Fat: 72%
Protein: 18%

INGREDIENTS
1½ cups quinoa
Freshly ground black pepper
1 teaspoon kosher salt
3 tablespoons fresh lemon juice
¼ cup olive oil, plus more
1 bunch scallions
1 pint cherry tomatoes
1 avocado, cut into 1-inch pieces
½ cup mint leaves
¼ cup chopped toasted pistachios
Sea Salt

INSTRUCTIONS
1. Bring quinoa, 1 tsp. kosher salt, and 3 cups water to a boil in a medium saucepan.
2. Cover, reduce heat to low, and simmer until quinoa is tender, 8–10 minutes.
3. Remove pan from heat and let sit 15 minutes. Fluff quinoa with a fork; transfer to a large bowl.
4. Whisk lemon juice and ¼ cup oil in a small bowl. D
5. Drizzle over warm quinoa and toss to coat; season with salt and pepper. Let it cool.

6. Prepare a grill for medium-high heat. Grill scallions and tomatoes in a grill basket, turning occasionally, until charred in spots and tomatoes begin to split, 6–8 minutes.
7. Transfer to a cutting board and slice scallions into 1" pieces.
8. Spoon quinoa onto a platter and top with scallions, tomatoes, avocado, mint, and pistachios.
9. Drizzle with oil and sprinkle with sea salt.

Day 6: Shredded Chicken Chili

Carbohydrates: 58%
Fat: 5%
Protein: 37%

INGREDIENTS
6 cups chicken stock
3 to 4 cups cooked shredded chicken
2 (15-ounce) cans beans of your choice, rinsed and drained (I used Great Northern beans)
2 cups (16 ounces) salsa verde
2 teaspoons ground cumin
optional toppings: diced avocado, chopped fresh cilantro, shredded cheese, chopped red or green onions, sour cream, crumbled tortilla chips

INSTRUCTIONS
1. Combine ingredients.
2. Stir together chicken stock, shredded chicken, beans, salsa and cumin in large stockpot.
3. Bring to a simmer.
4. Cook on high heat until the soup reaches a simmer. Then reduce heat to medium-low to maintain the simmer.
5. Serve.

Day 7: Shrimp Avocado Salad

Carbohydrates: 13%
Fat: 39%
Protein: 48%

INGREDIENTS
SALAD INGREDIENTS:
2 ears of sweet corn, shaved off the cob
3 strips of bacon, diced
1/2 lb. large shrimp, peeled with tails on or off
4 cups chopped Romaine lettuce
1 avocado, peeled, pitted and diced
1/3 cup grated Fontina cheese (optional)
buttermilk pesto dressing (see below)

BUTTERMILK PESTO DRESSING
INGREDIENTS:
1/2 cup buttermilk
1/2 cup mayo or Greek yogurt
1/4 cup pesto, homemade or store bought
1 small shallot, minced
1 Tbsp. lemon juice
pinch of salt and pepper, to taste

INSTRUCTIONS
TO MAKE THE SALAD:
1. Heat a skillet over high heat.
2. Add the corn kernels and let them dry-roast for about 6-8 minutes, stirring occasionally, until their edges begin to brown and caramelize.
3. Transfer the corn to a plate to set aside.

4. Reduce heat to medium-high. In the same skillet, add the bacon.
5. Fry for about 6 minutes, stirring occasionally, until crispy.
6. Remove the bacon with a slotted spoon, leaving the grease in the skillet.
7. Add the shrimp and saute until cooked and pink, about 2 minutes per side (depending on the size of your shrimp).
8. Remove shrimp and set aside.
9. Assemble your salads by tossing together the Romaine, corn, bacon, shrimp and avocado.
10. Drizzle with dressing and serve.

TO MAKE THE DRESSING:
1. Whisk together all ingredients until blended.
2. Season with salt and pepper.

References

8 Easy Steps to Kick Gluten to the Curb ... Permanently. (2020, April 7). Retrieved May 22, 2020, from https://www.verywellfit.com/how-to-go-gluten-free-563172

Akhondi, H. (2020, March 24). Gluten And Associated Medical Problems - StatPearls - NCBI Bookshelf. Retrieved May 2020, from https://www.ncbi.nlm.nih.gov/books/NBK538505/

Autoimmune disease. (2014, January 1). Retrieved May 2020, from https://www.sciencedirect.com/science/article/pii/B9780702054013000187

Autoimmune Disease List – AARDA. (2018). Retrieved May 18, 2020, from https://www.aarda.org/diseaselist/

Bell, M. B. S. (2017, February 2). Is Leaky Gut Syndrome a Real Condition? An Unbiased Look. Retrieved May 20, 2020, from https://www.healthline.com/nutrition/is-leaky-gut-real

Cohen, I., Day, A., & Shaoul, R. (2019, January 1). Gluten in Celiac Disease—More or Less? Retrieved May 17, 2020, from https://www.ncbi.nlm.nih.gov/pmc/articles/PMC6363368/

Day, L. (2011). Wheat gluten: production, properties and application. Retrieved 2020, from https://www.sciencedirect.com/science/article/pii/B9781845697587500101

Diag, P. B. (2018, April). What is zonulin? – Creative Diagnostics Blog. Retrieved May 2020, from https://www.creative-diagnostics.com/blog/index.php/what-is-zonulin/

Dietary management of dermatitis herpetiformis. - PubMed - NCBI. (1987, October). Retrieved May 19, 2020, from https://www.ncbi.nlm.nih.gov/pubmed/3662571

EatingWell. (2019, May 1). Starting a Gluten-Free Diet: A Guide for Beginners. Retrieved May 15, 2020, from http://www.eatingwell.com/article/288542/starting-a-gluten-free-diet-a-guide-for-beginners/

Fairweather, D., & Rose, N. (2004, November 1). Women and Autoimmune Diseases. Retrieved May 18, 2020, from https://www.ncbi.nlm.nih.gov/pmc/articles/PMC3328995/

Food labeling: gluten-free labeling of foods. Final rule. - PubMed - NCBI. (2013, August). Retrieved May 18, 2020, from https://www.ncbi.nlm.nih.gov/pubmed/23923139

Gluten Free Food List | IBS Diets. (n.d.-a). Retrieved May 15, 2020, from https://www.ibsdiets.org/ibs/gluten-free-food-list/

Gluten Free Food List | IBS Diets. (n.d.-b). Retrieved May 18, 2020, from https://www.ibsdiets.org/ibs/gluten-free-food-list/

Gluten-Free Foods. (n.d.-a). Retrieved May 2020, from https://celiac.org/gluten-free-living/gluten-free-foods/

Gluten-Free Foods. (n.d.-b). Retrieved May 18, 2020, from https://celiac.org/gluten-free-living/gluten-free-foods/

Hill, A. (2020, January 13). What Is Gluten? Definition, Foods, and Side Effects. Retrieved May 2020, from https://www.healthline.com/nutrition/what-is-gluten

Jones, A. (2017, May 1). The Gluten-Free Diet: Fad or Necessity? Retrieved May 18, 2020, from https://www.ncbi.nlm.nih.gov/pmc/articles/PMC5439366/

Mackay, I. (1998, January 1). Autoimmune Diseases. Retrieved May 18, 2020, from https://www.sciencedirect.com/science/article/pii/B0122267656000761

Niland, B., & Cash, B. (2018, February). Health Benefits and Adverse Effects of a Gluten-Free Diet in Non–Celiac Disease Patients. Retrieved May 2020, from https://www.ncbi.nlm.nih.gov/pmc/articles/PMC5866307/

Nutrient Recommendations: Dietary Reference Intakes (DRI). (n.d.). Retrieved May 18, 2020, from https://ods.od.nih.gov/Health_Information/Dietary_Reference_Intakes.aspx

Okada, H., Kuhn, C., Feillet, H., & Bach, J.-F. (2010, April 1). The 'hygiene hypothesis' for autoimmune and allergic diseases: an update. Retrieved May 16, 2020, from https://www.ncbi.nlm.nih.gov/pmc/articles/PMC2841828/

pubmeddev. (2012, February). Leaky gut and autoimmune diseases. - PubMed - NCBI. Retrieved May 2020, from https://www.ncbi.nlm.nih.gov/pubmed/22109896

pubmeddev. (2015). Molecular mimicry as a mechanism for food immune reactivities and autoimmunity. - PubMed - NCBI. Retrieved May 2020, from https://www.ncbi.nlm.nih.gov/pubmed/25599184

pubmeddev. (2017, August). Celiac Disease and Nonceliac Gluten Sensitivity: A Review. - PubMed - NCBI. Retrieved May 15, 2020, from https://www.ncbi.nlm.nih.gov/pubmed/28810029

Rakel, D. (2012). *Integrative Medicine: Expert Consult Premium Edition - Enhanced Online Features and Print (Rakel, Integrative Medicine)* (3rd ed.). Philadelphia, USA: Elsevier Saunders.

Reilly, N. (2016, August). The Gluten-Free Diet: Recognizing Fact, Fiction, and Fad. Retrieved May 17, 2020, from https://secure.jbs.elsevierhealth.com/action/cookieAbsent?code=null

Svensson, J., Sildorf, S. M., Pipper, C. B., Kyvsgaard, J. N., Bøjstrup, J., Pociot, F. M., ... Buschard, K. (2016). Potential beneficial effects of a gluten-free diet in newly diagnosed children with type 1 diabetes: a pilot study. *SpringerPlus*, *5*(1), 1–8. https://doi.org/10.1186/s40064-016-2641-3

The Beginners Guide to Going Gluten Free | Vida sin gluten. (n.d.). Retrieved May 23, 2020, from https://www.schaer.com/en-us/a/how-go-gluten-free-beginners

Watson, S. (2019, March 26). Autoimmune Diseases: Types, Symptoms, Causes, and More. Retrieved May 15, 2020, from https://www.healthline.com/health/autoimmune-disorders

What medicines and non-food products have gluten? (n.d.). Retrieved May 22, 2020, from https://www.webmd.com/digestive-disorders/celiac-disease/qa/what-medicines-and-nonfood-products-have-gluten

Zuvarox, T. (2020, January 8). Malabsorption Syndromes - StatPearls - NCBI Bookshelf. Retrieved May 19, 2020, from https://www.ncbi.nlm.nih.gov/books/NBK553 106/

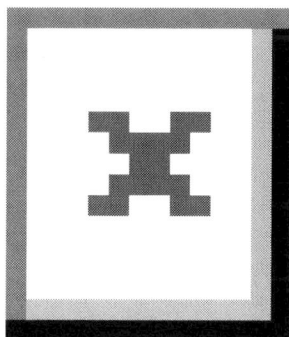

Printed in Great Britain
by Amazon